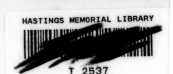

DATE DUE

SAFETY FIRST

Safety on the Go

Joanne Mattern
ABDO Publishing Company

visit us at
www.abdopub.com

Published by Abdo Publishing Company 4940 Viking Drive, Edina, Minnesota 55435.
Copyright © 1999 by Abdo Consulting Group, Inc. International copyrights reserved in all
countries. No part of this book may be reproduced in any form without written permission
from the publisher.

Printed in the United States.

Photo credits: Peter Arnold, Inc., Super Stock

Edited by Julie Berg
Contributing editor Morgan Hughes
Graphics by Linda O'Leary

Library of Congress Cataloging-in-Publication Data

Mattern, Joanne, 1963-
        Safety on the go / Joanne Mattern.
        p. cm. -- (Safety first)
        Includes index.
        Summary: Suggests how to be safe in situations involving transportation,
        including using safety belts, helping the driver stay safe, and practicing railroad
        safety.
        ISBN 1-57765-075-1
        1.Transportation--Safety measures--Juvenile literature. 2. Traffic safety--
        Juvenile literature. 3. Safety. [1. Transportation--Safety measures. 2. Safety.]
        I. Title. II. Series.
        HE 194.M38   1999
        363.12--dc21   21830

                                                                    98-17272
                                                                    CIP
                                                                    AC

Contents

Safety First! 4

Seat Belts for Safety 6

Safety in the Car 8

Helping the Driver Stay Safe 10

Waiting for Transportation 12

Railroad and Subway Safety 14

Boat Safety 16

Finding a Safe Seat 18

Staying Safe While You Ride 20

Glossary 22

Internet Sites 23

Index 24

Safety First!

There are lots of fun places to go every day! You go to school and your friends' houses. Or you might go to the museum or the park. To get to these places, you might ride in a car or a bus. Or you might take a train or subway.

No matter how you get where you're going, it is important to always stay safe. Staying safe means you won't get hurt. You won't get in trouble. And you will keep other people from getting hurt or in trouble, too!

How can you stay safe on public **transportation**? The best way is to follow the rules and think before you act. This book will show you many ways to put safety first when you are traveling.

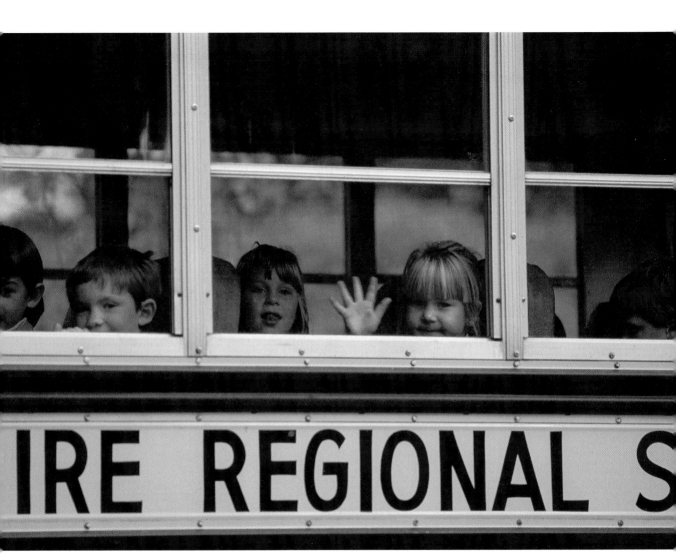

Sitting quietly on the bus is the safe way to ride.

Seat Belts for Safety

When you ride in a car, it's important to always wear your **seat belt**. A seat belt keeps you safe in case there is an **accident**. You should wear your seat belt even if you are just riding down the street or around the block.

Some cars have two seat belts. One is called a **shoulder belt**. This type of seat belt goes over your shoulder and across your body. The other type is a **lap belt**. It covers your hips. Be sure to wear both seat belts whenever you are in the car. They will work together to keep you safe.

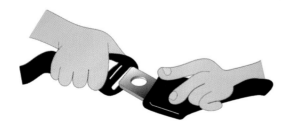

Listen for the click when you fasten your seat belt.

If your car has **air bags**, you should ride in the back seat. If you have to ride in the front, push the seat back as far as you can. That way, the air bag will have room to work without hurting you.

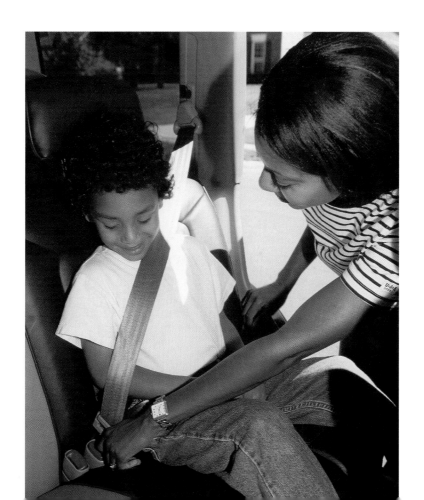

Safety in the Car

It's a good idea to keep all the doors locked while you are riding in a car. Locking the doors keeps you safe in two ways. It keeps bad people from breaking into your car. And it keeps you or other **passengers** from opening the door by **accident** while the car is moving. If the door opens while the car is moving, you might fall out! This won't happen if the door is locked and you are wearing your **seat belt**.

It's also safe to keep the car windows closed. Of course, when you get out of the car, make sure all the windows are closed and the doors are locked. Doing these things will keep your car safe!

This and opposite page: Keep the windows closed, the doors locked and your seat belt fastened to stay safe in the car.

8

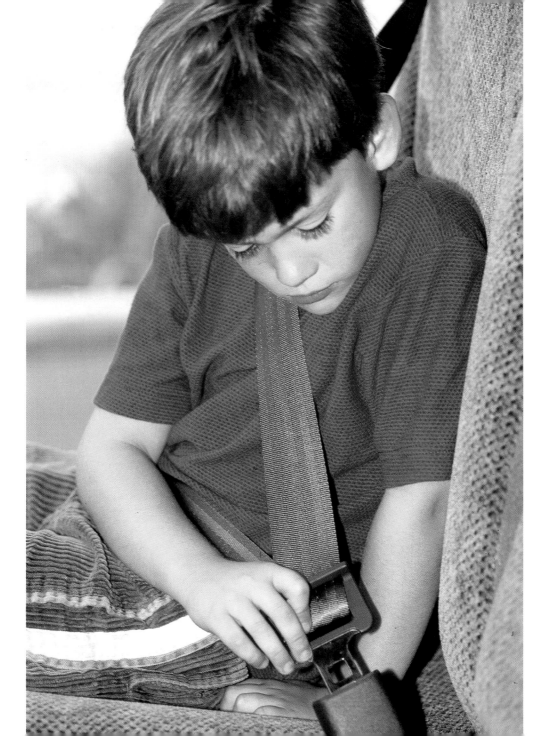

Helping the Driver Stay Safe

Driving a car might look easy, but it is hard work. There is a lot to think about. There is a lot to watch out for, too. The driver needs to pay attention to the road. That is why you should never bother the driver.

Don't move around or throw things in the car. Don't touch the driver or block his or her view. Shouting and fighting with other **passengers** or turning up the music too loud can distract the driver. Make sure you follow all the rules the driver asks you to.

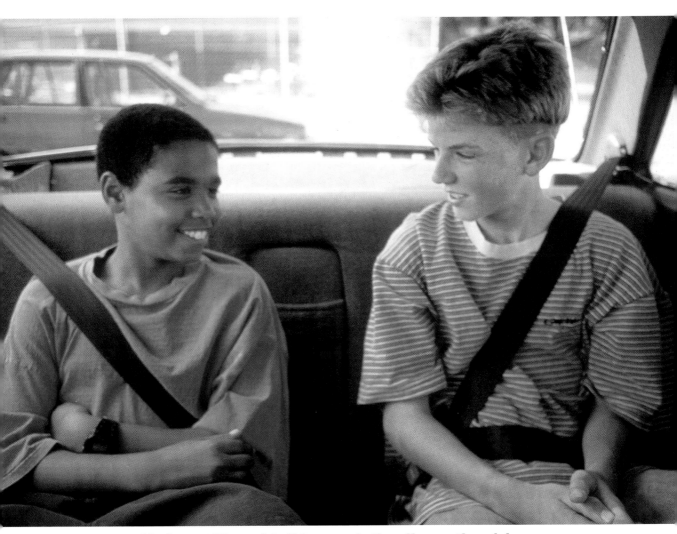

*Sitting still and talking quietly allows the driver
to pay attention to the road.*

Waiting for Transportation

Sometimes waiting for a bus or a train can be scary. There are ways to stay safe while waiting alone.

You should wait in a place where there is lots of light. Standing right under a street light is good. Avoid dark areas where people can't see you. It's better to wait out in the open. Don't stand near bushes or empty buildings.

It's a good idea to wait with other people you know. If there is a police officer in the area, ask him or her to stand with you.

Opposite page:
Waiting for transportation
is safer with a friend.

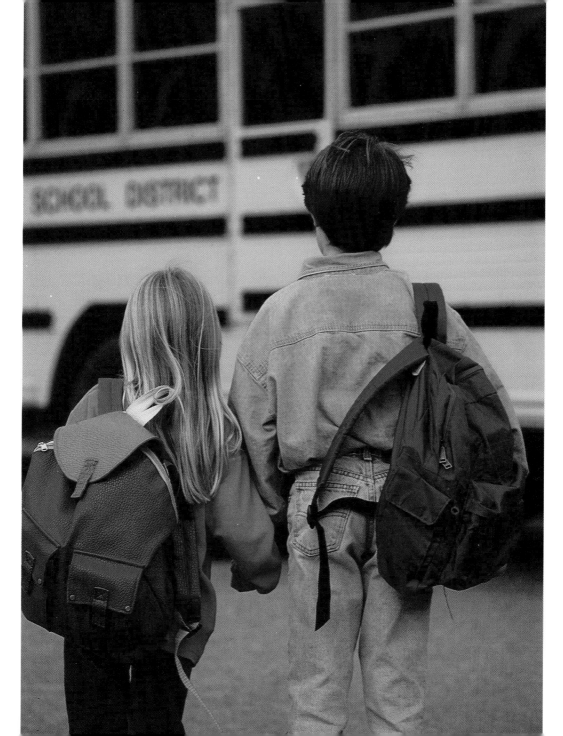

Railroad and Subway Safety

Never stand on the tracks when you are waiting for a train or a subway. Wait on the **platform** instead. If you have to cross the tracks, look both ways to make sure a train isn't coming. Listen for the train's whistle. Never run in front of a train.

When you are on the platform, be sure to stand away from the edge. There is usually a line painted along the edge of the platform. The safest place to wait is behind that line.

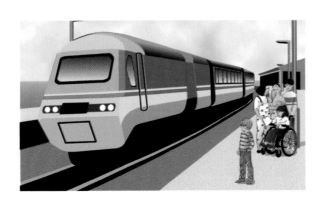

Stay on the platform when waiting for a train.

Subway tracks are even more **dangerous** than railroad tracks because they have a **third rail**. The third rail carries **electricity**. If you touch the third rail, you can get a bad **shock**.

When you are riding on the subway, don't walk from one car to another while the train is moving. It is not safe. The best way to stay safe is to stay seated.

Subway rails are dangerous because the third rail is electrified.

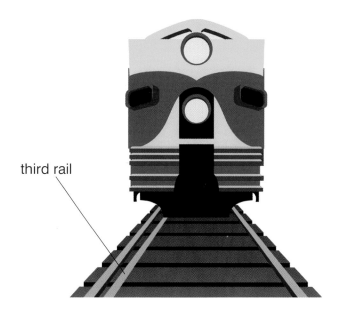

third rail

Boat Safety

Riding on a boat is fun, but it can also be **dangerous**. If you are riding on a small boat, be sure to wear a **life jacket**. This jacket will help you float if you fall in the water. In many states, the law says you have to wear a life jacket.

You don't have to wear a life jacket if you are on a large boat, such as a ferry or a cruise ship. But you still need to stay safe. Never hang over the railing or lean over the water. You might fall in!

You should also be careful walking around on a boat. The motion of the waves makes a boat rock up and down. This can make it hard to keep your balance. You should never run on a boat, either. It's easy to trip and fall—and that's not safe.

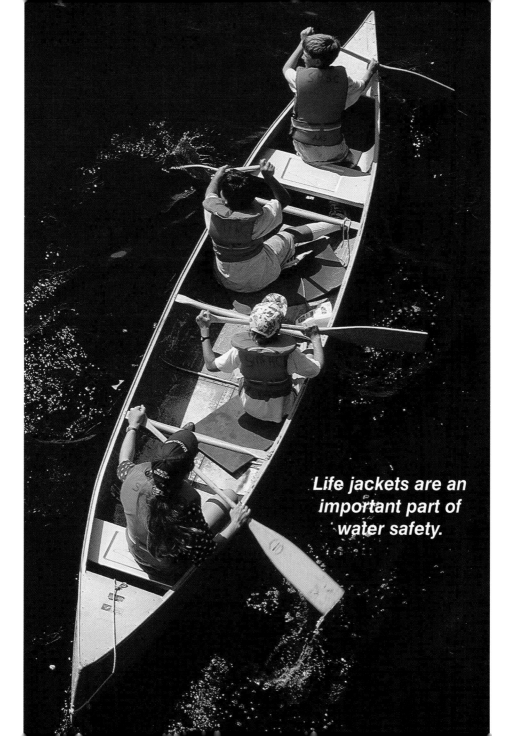

Life jackets are an important part of water safety.

Finding a Safe Seat

Once you get on the subway, bus, or train, you still need to put safety first. If you are on a bus, take a seat in the front, near the driver, if possible. If someone makes you feel scared, don't sit next to that person.

If you are riding on a train or subway, don't sit in a car by yourself. Find a car where other people are riding. Choose a seat next to people you think you can trust. Sitting next to a family is usually a good idea.

If you ride in an airplane by yourself, make sure that a flight attendant knows you are alone. Don't talk to strangers, even if they seem friendly. Tell the flight attendant if you feel scared.

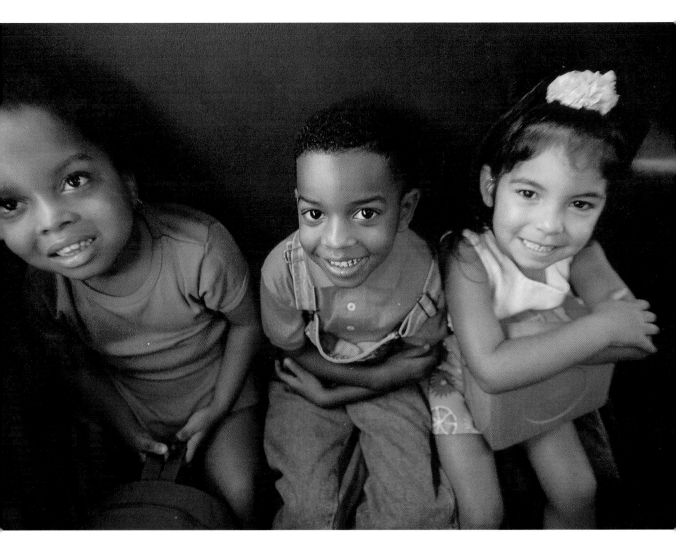

Sitting with a friend can make you feel safe.

Staying Safe While You Ride

The best way to stay safe on a bus or train is to sit down. If you walk around while the vehicle is moving, you might lose your balance and fall.

If you can't find a seat, hold onto something so you don't fall. Subway cars and buses have bars or straps for people to hang on to. You can also hold onto the back of a seat. Stay alert and think about keeping your balance. Be careful when the vehicle slows down or turns a sharp corner.

If you ride on an airplane, listen to all the safety rules that the flight attendants talk about at the beginning of the flight. Take off your **seat belt** only when you have to leave your seat. Sit quietly in your seat in case others are trying to sleep.

Remembering these simple rules is the best way to have fun on public **transportation**. To have a safe trip, always put safety first!

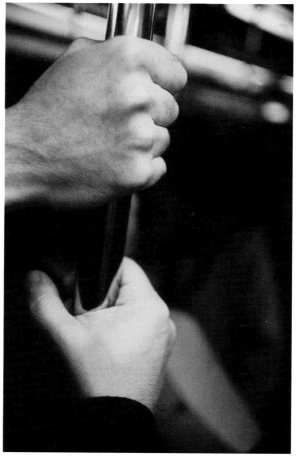

Hang onto a strap or pole if you can't find a seat.

Glossary

Accident (AK-si-duhnt) - something that takes place without planning it.

Air bag - in a car, a bag that inflates to protect a person in case of an accident.

Dangerous (DAYN-jur-uhss) - likely to cause harm; not safe.

Electricity (ih-lek-TRISS-uh-tee) - a form of energy.

Lap belt - a seat belt that crosses a person's lap.

Life jacket (life JAK-it) - a jacket that will keep you afloat in the water.

Passenger (PASS-uhn-jur) - someone besides the driver who travels in a car or other vehicle.

Platform (PLAT-form) - a flat, raised structure where people can stand.

Seat belt - a strap or harness that holds a person in the seat of a car, bus, train, or airplane in case of an accident.

Shock (SHOK) - the violent effect of an electric current passing through someone's body.

Shoulder belt (SHOHL-dur belt) - a seat belt that crosses the upper body.

Third rail - a metal rail that carries electric current to the motor of a subway.

Transportation (TRANS-pore-ta-shun) - traveling by bus, car, subway, train, or airplane. A way of getting from one place to another.

Internet Sites

Bicycling Safety
http://www.cam.org/~skippy/sites/cycling/SafetyLinks.html
Stories, studies, statistics, and tips on everything from safe cycling practices to maintenance. Special interest sections for kids and parents, and links to many interesting sites!

Safety Tips for Kids on the Internet
http://www.fbi.gov/kids/internet/internet.htm
The FBI has set up a "safety tips for the internet" website. It has very good information about how to protect yourself online.

National School Safety Center
http://www.nssc1.org/
This site provides training and resources for preventing school crime and violence.

Home Safety
http://www.safewithin.com/homesafe/
This site helps to make the home more secure, info on the health of the home environment and other safety resources.

These sites are subject to change.

Pass It On

Educate readers around the country by passing on information you've learned about staying safe. Share your little-known facts and interesting stories. Tell others about bike riding, school experiences, and any other stuff you'd like to discuss. We want to hear from you!

To get posted on the ABDO Publishing Company website E-mail us at
"adventure@abdopub.com"

Download a free screen saver at www.abdopub.com

Index

A

accident 6, 8
air bags 7
airplane 18, 20

B

boat safety 16
buildings 12
bus 4, 12, 18, 20

C

car 4, 6, 7, 8, 10,
  15, 18, 20

D

dangerous 15, 16
dark areas 12
driver 10, 18
driving 10

E

electricity 15

F

fighting 10
fun 4, 16, 21

L

lap belt 6
life jacket 16
locking the doors 8

M

museum 4

P

park 4
passenger 8, 10
platform 14
police officer 12
public transportation
  4, 21

R

railroad 15
rules 4, 10, 20, 21

S

school 4
seat belt 6, 8, 20
shoulder belt 6
shouting 10
street light 12
subway 4, 14, 15,
  18, 20

T

third rail 15
tracks 14, 15
train 4, 12, 14, 15,
  18, 20
transportation 4, 21
traveling 4

W

water 16
waves 16
windows 8